Final Report on Formaldehyde Levels

in FEMA-Supplied Travel Trailers, Park Models, and Mobile Homes

From the Centers for Disease Control and Prevention

July 2, 2008

Amended December 15th, 2010

Table of Contents

Final Report on Formaldehyde Levels
in FEMA-Supplied Travel Trailers, Park Models, and Mobile Homes

From the Centers for Disease Control and Prevention
July 2, 2008

EXECUTIVE SUMMARY

In December 2007 and January 2008, the Centers for Disease Control and Prevention (CDC) measured formaldehyde levels in a stratified random sample of 519 FEMA-supplied occupied travel trailers, park models, and mobile homes (i.e., "trailers"). At the time of the study, sampled trailers were in use as temporary shelter for Louisiana and Mississippi residents displaced by hurricanes Katrina and Rita. The study aimed to determine formaldehyde levels in occupied trailers, determine trailer characteristics that could affect formaldehyde levels, and provide information to assist FEMA in deciding whether to relocate residents from FEMA-supplied trailers in the Gulf Coast area. This study assessed only current formaldehyde levels in the occupied trailers; it was not a health effects study.

To evaluate levels of formaldehyde, investigators conducted a 1-hour continuous indoor air sample and sample measurements of indoor temperature and relative humidity. To determine factors that could affect formaldehyde levels, investigators administered a short questionnaire to adult residents about occupant demographics and trailer characteristics. To observe the exterior and interior of the trailer, investigators conducted a walk-through survey.

In many of the trailers tested, formaldehyde levels were higher than typical U.S. indoor levels. The geometric mean level of formaldehyde in sampled trailers was 77 ppb (range: 3–590 ppb). Formaldehyde levels varied by trailer type, but all types tested had some levels $\geq$ 100 ppb, the level at which health effects have been described in sensitive persons.

In this study, travel trailers had significantly higher average formaldehyde levels than did park models and mobile homes. A higher proportion of travel trailers than park models and mobile homes also had formaldehyde levels $\geq$ 100 ppb and $\geq$ 300 ppb. In multivariate analysis, factors such as temperature; relative humidity; trailer type and brand; opened windows, doors, and scuttles; and presence of mold ($\geq$ 1 ft^2) were significantly associated with formaldehyde levels.

Because formaldehyde levels tend to be higher in newly constructed trailers and during warmer weather, levels measured in this study are likely to underrepresent long-term exposures; many of these trailers are approximately 2 years old, and the study was conducted during the winter. In addition, the study did not evaluate any specific patterns of use with respect to specific types of trailers.

On the basis of the data reported here and in previous scientific reports and publications about adverse health effects associated with exposure to elevated formaldehyde levels,

CDC recommended that FEMA relocate Gulf Coast residents displaced by hurricanes Katrina and Rita and still living in trailers. Relocation priority should be given to occupants suffering symptoms potentially attributable to formaldehyde exposure and to vulnerable populations, such as children, elderly persons, and persons with chronic respiratory illnesses.

BACKGROUND

On August 28 and 29, 2005, Hurricane Katrina—a Category 4 storm—made landfall on the U.S. Gulf Coast between New Orleans, Louisiana (LA), and Mobile, Alabama. On September 24, 2008, Hurricane Rita—a Category 3 storm—made landfall along the Texas-Louisiana border, Many families evacuated from the U.S. Gulf Coast region returned later to find their homes severely damaged.

Starting in October 2005, the Federal Emergency Management Agency (FEMA) provided temporary housing along the Gulf Coast by supplying approximately 100,000 trailers (see box). In LA, more than 60% of trailers provided to residents were on private property. In Mississippi (MS), more than 78% of trailers were on private property. The remaining trailers in both states were in FEMA-designated trailer parks.

CDC Testing of Occupied Trailers

From December 21, 2007, to January 23, 2008, the Centers for Disease Control and Prevention (CDC) assessed levels of formaldehyde in indoor air of a random sample of occupied FEMA-supplied trailers. Formaldehyde testing was one of several actions CDC initiated in response to a July 13, 2007, request from FEMA to investigate concerns about formaldehyde in occupied FEMA trailers in LA and MS. This report details only the testing of occupied trailers for formaldehyde levels; it was not a health effects study.

**Definitions for Trailers Used by FEMA
for Gulf Coast Residents Displaced by Hurricanes Katrina and Rita**

- **Mobile homes** are manufactured homes wider than 8 feet or longer than 40 feet (for an area >320 ft^2). They are built on permanent chassis; contain plumbing, heating, air-conditioning, and electrical systems; and are designed for use as permanent dwellings. Mobile homes are defined and regulated by the U.S. Department of Housing and Urban Development (HUD).
- **Park models** are manufactured homes of 320–400 ft^2 administratively exempted from HUD formaldehyde standards. Park models may be regulated by transportation authorities and by manufacturer acceptance of a voluntary American National Standards Institute standard applying to their construction.
- **Travel trailers** are wheel-mounted trailers designed to provide temporary living quarters during periods of recreation, camping, or travel. Travel trailers generally have size limits, such as 8 feet wide and 40 feet long, for an area <320 ft^2. Travel trailers generally are considered vehicles rather than structures and are regulated by state transportation authorities rather than by housing authorities. Travel trailers have been used principally for short-term housing needs. They are placed on private sites while a homeowner's permanent residence is repaired or in group configurations primarily to support displaced renters.
- **Manufactured homes** include mobile homes and park models and are used to meet both short- and long-term disaster housing needs. Manufactured homes typically are placed on commercial pads or in group sites developed expressly for this purpose.
- **"Trailers"** in this report refers collectively to travel trailers, park models, and mobile homes.

Formaldehyde Levels in Residential Indoor Air

Formaldehyde in homes is a longstanding issue. Formaldehyde frequently is used in plywood, fiberboard, resins, glues, carpets, and several other construction components. In the past, formaldehyde also was used in insulation of many homes. In March 1982, the U.S. Consumer Product Safety Commission (CPSC) called for a ban on urea foam formaldehyde insulation (UFFI) (US CPSC, 1982). Although several commercial groups challenged this ban, citing greater formaldehyde exposure from carpets and other building materials, UFFI use had dropped precipitously by the mid 1980s. However, homes built before or around the UFFI ban still had this insulation.

The 1982 ban on UFFI contributed to the decreased levels of formaldehyde in more recent studies. Changes in the type of pressed wood products containing formaldehyde resins or glues also contributed to the decrease. In the past, pressed wood products often contained urea-formaldehyde resins. Today these resins are not as widely used. Instead, many pressed wood products are constructed with phenol-formaldehyde products (commonly known as exterior-grade products). Phenol-formaldehyde products emit much less formaldehyde (US EPA, 2007).

Temperature, relative humidity (RH), ventilation, and age of house also contribute to differences in measured formaldehyde levels. In longitudinal studies, formaldehyde emission rates were nearly constant over the first 8 months after construction, and then began to decline, suggesting that formaldehyde off-gassing continues for extended periods but decreases with the age of the home (Park and Ikeda, 2006). Studies also show that older homes have lower formaldehyde levels than do newer homes (Hodgson et al., 2000; Gordon et al., 1999).

A 1985 U.S. study investigated formaldehyde levels in different types of housing (Stock and Mendez, 1985). Formaldehyde levels in 38 conventional U.S. homes averaged 40 parts per billion (ppb), with highs of 140 ppb. Nineteen apartments and 11 condominiums had average formaldehyde levels of 80 ppb and 90 ppb, respectively, with highs of 290 ppb. A more recent study of new homes found geometric mean (GM) formaldehyde levels of 34 ppb in manufactured homes and 36 ppb in site-built homes (Hodgson et al., 2000). This study suggested that formaldehyde levels in conventional homes have decreased greatly since the 1980s, possibly because of decreased use of plywood paneling and reduced emissions from the composite wood products used.

The U.S. Environmental Protection Agency's National Human Exposure Assessment Survey found a median formaldehyde level of 17 ppb, with a high of 332 ppb, in 189 Arizona homes (Gordon et al., 1999). In a recent study of 184 single-family homes in three cities, Weisel et al. (2005) found mean formaldehyde levels of 3 ppb in outdoor ambient air; 17 ppb in home indoor air; and 16–25 ppb in trailers.

These studies indicate a trend. Even though all homes have some formaldehyde, levels generally seem to have decreased since the early 1980s. Lower ventilation rates in manufactured homes and greater ratios of surface area to volume may factor in this trend (US CPSC, 1997).

Health Effects

Symptoms from acute exposure to formaldehyde commonly manifest as irritation of the throat, nose, eyes, skin, and upper respiratory tract. This upper respiratory tract irritation can exacerbate symptoms of asthma and other respiratory illnesses (Main et al., 1983; Bracken et al., 1985; Kilburn et al., 1985; Imbus et al., 1985; Anderson et al., 1979; Garret et al,. 1999[1]; Hendrick and Lane, 1977[1]; Institute of Medicine, 2000[1]; Jaakkola et al., 2004[1]; Kryzanowski et al., 1990[1]; McCoy, 2008[1]; NHLBI et al., 2007[1]; Nordman et al., 1985[1]; Rumchev et al., 2002[1]; Staab et al., 2008[1]; Thompson and Grafstrom, 2008[1]).

Acute and chronic health effects of exposure to formaldehyde vary by individual. At 800 ppb, nearly everyone develops some acute irritative symptoms; however, formaldehyde-sensitive persons have reported symptoms at levels around 100 ppb (Main et al., 1983; Bender et al., 1983; Hanrahan et al., 1984[1]). Additional studies have found health effects at 100 ppb in sensitive persons chronically exposed to formaldehyde (Ritchie et al., 1987; ATSDR 2010[1]). Typically olfactory recognition occurs around 500 ppb, leaving the average exposure from a home below this level. Sensitive and sensitized persons can experience symptoms without detecting odor and thus receive little or no warning of exposure (Kulle et al. 1987; Weisel et al. 2005; Fischer et al., 1995[1]; Garrett et al., 1999[1]; Kiec-Swierczynska, 1996[1]; Lee et al., 1984[1]; Maibach, 1983[1]; Marks et al., 1998[1]; Wantke and Wantke., 1996[1]).

In addition to acute health effects from formaldehyde, chronic effects in occupational settings have been studied. A study of 186 male plywood workers associated formaldehyde exposure with several respiratory symptoms, including cough and chronic bronchitis, and suggested that formaldehyde exposure induces symptoms of chronic obstructive lung disease (Malaka and Kodama, 1990). Funeral home workers reported chronic bronchitis more frequently than did controls who were not occupationally exposed to formaldehyde (Holness, 1989).

However, studies attempting to correlate worker-reported symptoms, such as cough or shortness of breath, with formal objective pulmonary function testing have shown conflicting results. Two studies demonstrated a small and reversible decrease in forced expiratory volume and forced vital capacity (Alexandersson et al., 1989; Alexandersson et al., 1982). Additional studies employing formal pulmonary function testing demonstrated no significant difference in pulmonary function testing parameters (Horvath, 1988; Holness et al., 1989).

The carcinogenicity of formaldehyde has been extensively studied during the last 30 years. In June 2004, the International Agency for Research on Cancer (IARC) reclassified formaldehyde from "probably carcinogenic to humans" to "carcinogenic to humans." IARC has concluded that formaldehyde exposure causes nasopharyngeal cancer (http://monographs.iarc.fr/ENG/Meetings /88-formaldehyde.pdf). However, the National Institutes of Health National Toxicology Program has not adopted IARC's classification change and continues to classify formaldehyde as "reasonably anticipated to be a carcinogen in humans" (http://ntp.niehs.nih.gov/ntp/roc/eleventh/profiles/s089form.pdf).

---

[1] CDC added this reference on December 15, 2010 in response to an Information Request for Correction (http://aspe hhs.gov/infoquality/request&response/35b8.pdf)

How to quantitatively relate measured air levels of formaldehyde to cancer risk is uncertain. Because many other factors play a role in the development of cancer and because formaldehyde is ubiquitous in the environment, no definitive level can be established that places humans in a "high-risk" category. The safest way to reduce risk for cancer is to limit exposure. Clinically useful biologic markers, such as blood or urine tests, also are lacking, further complicating the ability to link exposure with outcome. Because formaldehyde plays integral physiologic roles and has a short half-life in the body, determining what is necessary for normal physiologic function and what is excessive and potentially harmful is difficult (Sullivan and Kreiger, 2001; Baselt, 1994). In general, the lower the level and shorter the duration of exposure, the lower the risk for cancer and other health effects.

Regulations and Standards of Formaldehyde Levels
No federal regulation or standard exists for formaldehyde levels in residential settings. Occupational levels are not appropriate to apply to residential settings for a variety of reasons. For example, residential populations include children and elderly persons and thus are more diverse than occupational populations and possibly more susceptible to illness from exposure because of preexisting health conditions. Exposure times and circumstances in homes can vary substantially from those in occupational settings. Many occupational settings have ongoing monitoring programs and may have safety requirements to reduce formaldehyde exposure (US Department of Labor, 2007). Even for workers, regulations and standards established for formaldehyde by government agencies and other organizations—such as the Occupational Safety and Health Administration, CDC's National Institute for Occupational Safety and Health, and the American Conference of Governmental Industrial Hygienists—differ markedly for both long- and short-term exposures (Federal Register, 1992; NIOSH, 1992; ACGIH, 1993).

Various nonoccupational standards also vary The U.S. Department of Housing and Urban Development (HUD) regulates formaldehyde emissions from wood products used in the construction of manufactured housing. HUD's maximum allowed levels for formaldehyde emissions from wood products are 200 ppb for plywood and 300 ppb for particle board (http://ecfr.gpoaccess.gov). The World Health Organization guideline for formaldehyde in nonoccupational settings is 100 ppb for 30 minutes. This guideline was developed to protect against sensory irritation in the general population, but it also represents an exposure level at which risk for upper respiratory tract cancer in humans is negligible (WHO, 1989). The State of California Office of Environmental Health Hazard Assessment (OEHHA) guideline for formaldehyde is less than typical ambient levels, it recommended an office level of 23 ppb (http://www.oehha.ca.gov/air/chronic_rels/AllChrels.html).

OBJECTIVES

The objectives of this study were to
1. Determine formaldehyde levels in occupied trailers.
2. Determine factors or characteristics of occupied trailers—not specific to any particular type of trailer—that could affect formaldehyde levels.
3. Provide information to assist FEMA in making decisions about relocating residents from FEMA-supplied trailers still used in the Gulf Coast area.

METHODS

To evaluate the formaldehyde levels and to determine potential factors and characteristics of occupied trailers that can impact formaldehyde levels, study investigators collected the following data for each participating trailer:

- A 1-hour, time-integrated indoor sample measurement of formaldehyde.
- A concurrent sample measurement of indoor temperature and RH
- A short questionnaire administered to adult residents to obtain demographic information about trailer residents and typical daily activities.
- A short walk-through survey to assess the indoor environment and the home exterior.

Study Personnel

Staff who collected the data were contractors from Bureau Veritas (Kennesaw, GA). Their training at the beginning of the study included review of recruitment, data collection, trailer visits, data records, and the protocol. CDC staff monitored contract staff throughout the study and were always available for consultation.

Trailer Selection

Using disproportionate stratified random sampling, CDC investigators selected 519 trailers for participation from a FEMA-provided list of 46,970 trailers in LA and MS that were identified as occupied as of November 2007. SAS 9.1 was used to randomly generate a list of sample trailers.

The three trailer types most commonly used—travel trailer, park model, and mobile home—were divided into a total of 11 strata. Travel trailers comprised seven strata: the top six manufacturers (Gulfstream, Forest River, Fleetwood, Fleetwood CA, Pilgrim, and Keystone [which together represented 61% of occupied travel trailers]) and "all other" travel-trailer brands. Because Gulfstream was the most frequently used travel trailer, that brand was oversampled. Park models comprised two strata: the most common model manufactured by Silver Creek (21% of park models) and "all other" park model manufacturers. Mobile homes also comprised two strata: the most common model manufactured by Cavalier (17% of mobile homes used) and "all other" manufacturers. Each brand in the "all other" groups made up <3% of the trailers.

The number of trailers selected was based on power calculations that allow researchers to draw statistically valid conclusions about the population of occupied trailers studied (i.e., FEMA-supplied trailers used) and for common trailer types and brands within that population of FEMA-supplied trailers. With a level of significance of 5% (95% confidence) and power of 80%, the goal was to sample a minimum of 38 trailers to detect an average difference of 30 ppb for each stratum. Sample sizes were calculated as tests for each stratum mean against the mean for the entire sample.

Within each stratum, each trailer was assigned a random number (e.g., SAS: Randval=randuni[number]). Each list then was sorted in numeric order according to the random number assignment. In recruiting eligible households, investigators followed a specific protocol (Appendix A) and used these ordered active call lists to recruit participants for the study, beginning with number 1 and ending with number 120 for the Gulfstream stratum and with number 38 for each of the other 10 strata. When the occupant of a selected trailer could not be contacted, declined participation, or was ineligible, investigators called the next trailer on the list, adding trailers as necessary from a reserve list, until they had successfully enrolled 120 trailers in the Gulfstream stratum and 38 trailers in each of the other 11 strata.

Up to three telephone numbers were provided for each trailer. Over a 1-week period, investigators attempted a total of 15 times separate attempts to contact a selected trailer. The 15 attempts included various times of the day and days of the week. If unsuccessful after 15 attempts, the trailer was moved to the "unable to contact" list and a new trailer from the reserve list was added to the active call list.

Contract staff followed a phone script (Appendix B) when speaking with the self-identified adult resident and recorded each attempt in a phone log (Appendix B). If the adult resident of an eligible household agreed to participate, a time was scheduled to conduct the sampling. If the adult resident declined to participate, the trailer was moved to the "refused to participate" list and a new trailer from the reserve list was added to the active call list.

Some enrolled households were expected to not complete the study for a variety of reasons. Each time it was determined that an enrolled trailer was to be removed from the list of participants, a new trailer from the reserve list was substituted and recruitment procedures as described above were followed.

Eligibility Criteria
Adult residents who agreed to participate were enrolled in the study. Eligibility criteria for participation in the study specified that:

- The consenting adult resident was ≥ 18 years of age.

- The adult resident resided in a FEMA-issued trailer in MS or LA at the time of phone recruitment.

- The adult resident reported that he or she spent at least 6 hours each day in a FEMA-issued trailer.

- The adult resident agreed to participate.

Consent/Assent Process

Adult residents provided informed assent (Appendix C) which was first obtained from the contacted adult resident during the scripted recruitment phone call. A second informed consent form was provided to the participant and signed in person sample collection (Appendix D). All participants received appropriate notification of confidentiality. CDC's Institutional Review Board reviewed and approved this study (CDC Protocol #5320, approved by CDC IRB-G on December 20, 2007).

Variables

The primary outcome variable was the 1-hour average level of formaldehyde measured in the air of occupied trailers. To determine potential factors of occupied trailers that can affect the measured formaldehyde levels, other variables were collected during an exposure assessment and walk-through.

Exposure Assessment Questionnaire

Investigators administered a short questionnaire (Appendix E) to the adult resident during the 1-hour sample collection process. The questionnaire inquired about the demographics of the trailer occupants and the average number of hours spent inside and outside the trailer. It also inquired about factors that can influence the indoor environment of the trailer, such as occupant smoking and frequency of air conditioning, heating, and window use. Daily and recent activities in the trailer, such as cooking, also were recorded.

Environmental Walk-Through Survey

During the walk-through survey (Appendix E), investigators surveyed the interior and exterior of the trailer, observing such factors as holes and leaks, mold, type of cooking fuel, and working smoke detectors.

Formaldehyde Sample Collection

Investigators and FEMA field workers were present for each scheduled sampling appointment. Investigators collected a 1-hour sample of air in each participating trailer using the NIOSH Manual of Analytical Methods Method 2016 using Supelco S10 LpDNPH cartridges (St. Louis, MO) (http://www.cdc.gov/niosh/nmam/pdfs/2016.pdf). Staff also measured indoor temperature and RH. In an attempt to standardize living conditions between trailers, residents were asked to configure doors and windows as they would have them while they slept. No cooking or smoking was allowed in the travel trailers or mobile homes during the 1-hour sample collection period because these activities could affect formaldehyde levels.

Samples were collected using standard industrial hygiene pumps. Samples were drawn at a flow rate of 500 ± 50 mL per minute for 1 hour at a height of 4 feet, which is comparable to a person's breathing zone while sitting. An investigator observed sample collection at all times. Investigators followed all quality assurance and quality control standards as outlined in the standard operating procedures for field collection (Appendix F).

Samples were analyzed for formaldehyde levels at the Bureau Veritas laboratory in Novi, Michigan. The Bureau Veritas laboratory is a contract laboratory for NIOSH and follows NIOSH data quality objectives in its sampling and analysis.

Temperature and Relative Humidity Sample Collection

A concurrent 1-hour reading of temperature and RH was collected in the center of the trailer primary living room using a HOBO® temperature and RH logging instrument manufactured by Onset Computer Corporation (Bourne, MA). The instrument collected data at 5-minute intervals. Data were collected for a minimum of 70 minutes, beginning at least 5 minutes before and lasting at least 5 minutes after collection of the formaldehyde sample at each trailer.

Sample Collection Data Sheet
Investigators completed a data sheet (Appendix G) for formaldehyde, temperature, and RH. Information included sample start and finish time, location of sample collection, and flow calibration results before and after sample collection was recorded. The data sheet accompanied the questionnaire and the walk-through survey (Appendix E).

Data Collection, Entry, Editing, and Management
Investigators collected all questionnaire, survey, and field data; labeled all samples and documentation with a unique alphanumeric identifier; and logged all paperwork and samples as they completed each trailer. Strict quality assurance and quality control procedures were observed.

Investigators entered all field data into an electronic database. All participant information remained confidential and was used only for the study. Access to data was restricted to those involved in conducting the study. In addition, all reports—published and internal—were based only on aggregate data. Investigators returned or destroyed all data sources after delivering the final approved database to CDC.

Statistical Analysis
All statistical analyses were conducted using SAS 9.1. The SURVEYMEANS, SURVEYREG, and SURVEYFREQ procedures were used to account for the stratified sampling design. Unweighted frequencies of questionnaire items were calculated using the FREQ procedure.

Data were examined and potential misclassifications of trailers resolved. The manufacturer, manufacturer's vehicle identification number, and trailer type were examined to confirm the categorization of each trailer. In cases where a trailer was recategorized, two independent evaluators agreed on the new classification.

A natural log transformation was applied to the formaldehyde levels to normalize the distribution. Tests for normality were conducted on the transformed levels, and the levels were plotted to examine the form of the distribution. Univariate linear regression models were constructed to evaluate the significance of selected questionnaire items in predicting the natural log of formaldehyde levels. Variables with cell counts of five or fewer were not included in the regression models.

Temperature and RH were evaluated separately as both continuous and categorical variables. Recorded signs of mold in the living area of the trailer were used to create a dichotomous variable indicating whether the trailer had <1 ft^2 of mold versus ≥ 1 ft^2 of mold.

Because the SAS SURVEYREG procedure does not include an option for automated model selection, CDC staff manually performed a backward elimination procedure. All independent variables with cell counts greater than five initially were entered into the linear regression model. At each step, the variable contributing the least to the model, as assessed by the F statistic, was removed. The final model included variables that were significant at a P of ≤ 0.05.

RESULTS

Participation Rates

During recruitment, investigators contacted residents at 1137 (76%) of the 1489 trailers on the FEMA-supplied list (Figure 1). Of the 717 eligible trailers, occupants in 519 (72%) participated. Reasons for ineligibility of the remaining 420 trailers included trailer not occupied (367 [87%]); trailer type no longer needed for its stratum (27 [6%]); trailer occupant unable to schedule an appointment time because of work, travel, hospitalization, or other reasons (15 [4%]); hostility by occupants (3 [1%]); and unknown reasons (8 [2%]).

Most trailers sampled were in LA and were located on private land (Table 1). Most were issued in 2005 and therefore were at least 2 years old at the time of testing. Seventy-seven percent of total occupants were adults. Recategorization of trailers resulted in reclassification of 35 trailers (7%) to new strata. The majority of these reclassified trailers came from the nonspecific "other" strata.

Overall Range and Variability of Formaldehyde Levels

The geometric mean (GM) formaldehyde level for all trailers sampled was 77 ppb (95% confidence interval [CI]: 70–85; range: 3–590 ppb). Throughout this report, when mean formaldehyde levels are discussed they will refer to GM formaldehyde levels. The GM formaldehyde level was 81 ppb for travel trailers (95% CI: 72–92), 44 ppb for park models (95% CI: 38–53) and 57 ppb for mobile homes (95% CI: 49–65) (Figure 2). GM formaldehyde levels varied significantly among travel trailers, park models, and mobile homes ($P < 0.001$) and ranged widely in all types of trailers. In all three trailer types, some trailers had formaldehyde levels $\geq$ 100 ppb. Mobile homes and travel trailers each had levels $\geq$ 300 ppb (Table 2). GM formaldehyde levels differed significantly among strata, but each stratum included some trailers with levels $\geq$ 100 ppb (Table 3).

Occupant Activities

The investigation included occupant activities in the trailers (Table 4). Air conditioning was used <4 hours per day in 71%; heat was used <4 hours a day in 56%; and space heaters were used in 44%. For 34% of trailers, residents reported someone had smoked in the trailer within 2 weeks before the sampling. Eighty-one percent of respondents cooked in their trailers. Pets were present in 25% of trailers, with dogs (20%) most commonly reported. More than 80% of respondents spent >8 hours in their trailer each day.

Occupant activities directly preceding the sampling period were recorded to determine whether they significantly affected sampling results. Within 3 hours before testing, 44% of homes had windows, doors, and scuttles open, and smoking had occurred in 19%. Other activities in the week before testing included use of air fresheners (61%); candles (24%); and glue, paint, or furniture finish (3%). These finding did not correlate with any specific type of trailer.

Trailer Characteristics

Specific characteristics of each sampled trailer were recorded. Respondents reported roof leaks in 17% of trailers, pipe leaks in 15%, and mold in 21%.

Walk-Through Survey
On the day of sampling, investigators walked through each trailer to record specific characteristics and information (Table 5). Propane gas was the most commonly used fuel for cooking (71% of trailers). Six percent of trailers had at least 1 ft^2 of mold. Twenty-nine percent of trailers did not have a functioning smoke detector.

Multivariate Analysis
Backward elimination modeling yielded a final regression model containing the following statistically significant variables: stratum ($P < 0.0001$); average temperature in degrees F ($P < 0.0001$); RH expressed as a percentage ($P < 0.0001$); a dichotomous variable indicating whether doors, windows, or scuttles were open in the 3 hours before testing ($P = 0.02$); and a dichotomous variable indicating the amount of mold observed in the trailer (≥ 1 ft^2) ($P = 0.05$). The dependent variable was the natural log of the formaldehyde levels. Temperature accounted for the most variation in the natural log of formaldehyde levels explained by the model (Figures 3 and 4) show the unadjusted relationship between the natural log of formaldehyde and temperature and humidity, respectively. Temperature ranged from 41°F to 91°F, and RH was 23%–88%.

Temperature and RH were evaluated separately as both continuous and categorical variables. Results were similar, so investigators included the continuous variables in the final model. Interactions between independent variables were not significant.

The presence of ≥ 1 ft^2 of mold was associated with a significant increase in GM formaldehyde levels (adjusted mean 86 ppb versus 63 ppb) (Table 6). Windows, doors, or scuttles open in the 3 hours before testing was associated with a significant decrease in GM formaldehyde levels (adjusted mean 65 ppb versus 83 ppb) (Table 7). Although each of three strata (Forest River, other park models, and other mobile homes) contained fewer than 38 trailers, contrasts comparing the GM formaldehyde level in each of them to the overall GM of the others still showed significant differences ($P = 0.01$, 0.01, and 0.04, respectively).

GM formaldehyde levels in travel trailers manufactured by Fleetwood and Fleetwood CA were significantly lower than levels in the other travel trailers combined, after adjustment for covariates ($P < 0.001$ for both). They did not differ significantly from each other. GM formaldehyde levels for Pilgrim, Keystone, and Gulfstream were significantly higher than for the other travel trailers combined, after adjustment for covariates ($P<0.001$ for all three). They did not differ significantly from each other. After adjustment for covariates, levels in Silver Creek park models were significantly lower than those in other park models ($P = 0.004$), and levels in Cavalier mobile homes were significantly higher than those in other mobile homes ($P = 0.006$). Table 8 presents the adjusted GM formaldehyde level by stratum from the multivariate model.

The parameter estimates (Table 9) can be used to calculate predicted formaldehyde levels. However, extrapolating beyond observed levels is not recommended. As an example, a Keystone travel trailer with an average temperature of 65°F; an average RH of 45%; no open doors, windows, or scuttles in the 3 hours before testing; and mold (≥ 1 ft^2) would have a predicted formaldehyde level of 88.5 ppb:

Natural log of formaldehyde = 0.012 + 0.096 + 65(0.052) + 45(0.017) +0(-0.243) + 0.311
Predicted formaldehyde: 88.5 ppb

DISCUSSION

Formaldehyde levels in the trailers in this study were higher than average levels in U.S. mobile homes and traditional homes reported in recent studies (Weisel et al., 2005; Gordon et al., 1999). As the formaldehyde level rises, risk for health consequences presumably also rises. At higher levels, people can have acute symptoms, such as coughing and irritated eyes, nose, throat, and upper respiratory system. Even at levels too low to cause such symptoms, risk for cancer can increase. No specific level of formaldehyde separates "safe" from "dangerous," especially in regard to cancer.

In this study, certain human activities were associated with higher formaldehyde levels. Open windows, doors, or scuttles decreased formaldehyde levels, indicating ventilation of trailers is an important recommendation to occupants. Keeping windows, doors, or scuttles open and the using air conditioning were associated with decreased levels of formaldehyde in trailers in a previous study (ATSDR, 2007). Yet many trailer air conditioners recirculate air and do not provide outside ventilation. Thus, less use of air conditioning may indicate increased ventilation because doors, windows, and scuttles are more likely to be open. Results of this study show a low use of air conditioning during the study period. Most trailers had working air conditioning, but most people did not use it more than 4 hours each day, most likely because the study was conducted during the winter; other factors could include cost and noise.

Smoking by occupants, though not significantly associated with increased formaldehyde levels in the multivariate analysis, was common and remains an important issue because cigarettes are a source of formaldehyde. Cigarette smoke also contains a wide range of other toxic and irritating compounds associated with increased health risk that can worsen air quality in the trailers.

The presence of mold ($\geq$ 1 ft^2) (6% of trailers) was associated with higher formaldehyde levels. Mold also can contribute to decreased indoor air quality and cause respiratory symptoms.

Cooking, particularly without outdoor-venting range hoods, can affect formaldehyde levels. The unvented combustion from gas-fired stoves can be a source of formaldehyde and other air pollutants and can increase the temperature and RH inside the trailer.

Increased indoor temperature and RH were associated with increased formaldehyde levels. These associations indicate exposure risks could increase during the summer, perhaps dramatically, with warmer and more humid weather. Formaldehyde levels during the winter may not represent summer levels.

Stratification was conducted to assess the possibility of an elevated formaldehyde level in one brand or a group of brands. Some brands showed higher GM formaldehyde levels than others, although this study showed all brands with some trailers $\geq$ 100 ppb, levels at which health effects have been described in sensitive persons. Formaldehyde levels varied by trailer type, but all types tested had some levels $\geq$ 100 ppb (Ritchie et al., 1987; Main et al., 1983; Bender et al., 1983).

LIMITATIONS

Study results are not representative of trailers purchased and used in other places and other situations because the sample for this study was selected only from occupied FEMA-supplied trailers in LA and MS. Formaldehyde levels in other trailers used elsewhere could differ by age, characteristics of manufacture, circumstances of use, or characteristics of environment.

Formaldehyde levels are expected to be lower in cooler temperatures and lower RH because of the processes of formaldehyde off-gassing. Therefore, levels measured in this study are likely to underestimate past levels—when trailers were hotter and more humid—and future levels— during summer months. Many of these trailers were >2 years old, and previous studies have shown highest formaldehyde levels in newer trailers and homes (Hodgson et al., 2000; Gordon et al., 1999), so residents were probably exposed to higher levels of formaldehyde when their trailers were newer.

Formaldehyde was measured at a central location in the trailer, and different locations in the trailer could have different formaldehyde levels. However, as a gas, formaldehyde is likely to diffuse evenly throughout the trailer. The results of this study do not apply to trailers used in other places and situations because this representative sample was selected only from FEMA-supplied trailers in LA and MS. This study does not assess the health status of people currently living in FEMA trailers, but further studies are planned to investigate potential health effects from living in trailers.

CONCLUSIONS
1. In many trailers tested, formaldehyde levels were higher than typical U.S. indoor levels.
2. The average level of formaldehyde in all trailers was 77 ppb, and many trailers had higher levels (range: 3 ppb–590 ppb) . These are higher than U.S. background levels, and occupant health could be affected at the levels recorded in many trailers.
3. These measured levels probably underrepresent occupant exposures in the early months of occupation and even the average exposure over time the trailers were occupied because formaldehyde levels tend to be higher in newly constructed trailers and during warm weather.
4. Higher indoor temperatures and RH were associated with higher formaldehyde levels in this study, independent of trailer type or brand.
5. Formaldehyde levels varied by trailer type, but all types tested had some levels $\geq$ 100 ppb, at which acute health effects can occur in sensitive persons.
6. Travel trailers had significantly higher average formaldehyde levels than park models or mobile homes. Travel trailers also had higher proportions of trailers with formaldehyde levels $\geq$ 100 and $\geq$ 300 ppb than park models or mobile homes.
7. Because some types and brands had lower average formaldehyde levels, trailers might be able to be manufactured or used in ways that reduce levels. Additional studies are under way to address this possibility.
8. Factors such as temperature; RH; closed windows, doors, and scuttles; and presence of

mold (≥ 1 ft^2) were associated with increased formaldehyde levels in the trailers. These were not assessed with respect to any specific type of trailer.

9. Only 71% of trailers sampled had a working smoke detector. Education is needed about the need for smoke detectors in the trailers and testing to ensure they function correctly.

RECOMMENDATIONS
Recommendations for Public Health, Emergency Response, and Housing Officials

1. These conclusions support decisions made need to relocate residents of the U.S. Gulf Coast region displaced by hurricanes Katrina and Rita who still live in trailers move quickly before temperatures in the region increased. On the basis of observations and previous scientific literature, priority should be given as follows:
   a. Persons currently experiencing symptoms possibly attributable to formaldehyde exposure,

   b. Especially vulnerable persons (e.g., children, the elderly, and those with chronic diseases), and
   c. Persons living in trailer types that tend to have higher formaldehyde levels.
2. Follow-up will require collaboration among multiple agencies—including FEMA, HUD, CDC, and state and local officials—to achieve safe, healthy housing for people displaced by hurricanes Katrina and Rita who continue to live in FEMA-supplied trailers.
3. Follow-up will require multiagency collaboration involving HUD, CDC, and others to assess the potential for formaldehyde levels in trailers used in other places and contexts, including trailers used for recreation, permanent housing, schools, and offices.
4. Federal, state, and local officials should consider how best to provide necessary assistance to the Louisiana and Mississippi state health departments to ensure adequate follow-up, including medical needs, for residents with health and medical concerns resulting from formaldehyde exposure while residing in FEMA-provided travel trailers, park models, and mobile homes.
5. Federal, state, and local officials should consider supporting establishment of a registry of people who resided in FEMA-supplied trailers in the U.S. Gulf Coast region.

Recommendations for Residents Awaiting Relocation
1. Spend as much time as possible outdoors in fresh air.
2. Open windows, doors, and scuttles as often as possible to let in fresh air.
3. Try to maintain the temperature inside trailers at the lowest comfortable level.
4. Do not smoke, especially not inside.
5. If you have health concerns, see a doctor or another medical professional.
6. All of these recommendations apply particularly to families with children, elderly persons, and those with chronic diseases, such as asthma.

Further CDC Action
1. CDC notified participants about their study results by personal visits from members of the U.S. Public Health Service Commissioned Corps and FEMA representatives and by hand-delivered letters.
2. At a series of 14 public availability sessions in LA and MS, CDC staff were available to talk with concerned and interested persons, provide information, and answer questions.

3. CDC is assessing formaldehyde levels across different models and types of unoccupied trailers to identify factors that decrease or increase those levels. This assessment also involves identifying cost-effective ways to reduce formaldehyde levels in trailers.
4. CDC is developing a protocol for a long-term health study, with a respiratory focus, of children who resided in FEMA trailers and mobile homes in LA and MS.
5. CDC provided educational materials and information to trailer residents about their risk for exposure to formaldehyde and ways to improve indoor air quality and health.
6. CDC reconvened a panel of experts on this issue to identify and provide input on health issues potentially associated with long-term residence in trailers.

REFERENCES

[ATSDR] Agency for Toxic Substances and Disease Registry. 2007. An Update and Revision of ATSDR's February 2007 Health Consultation: Formaldehyde Sampling of FEMA Temporary-Housing Trailers, Baton Rouge, Louisiana, September–October 2006. [cited October 2007]. Available from: http://www.atsdr.cdc.gov.

[ATSDR] Agency for Toxic Substances and Disease Registry. (1999). "Formaldehyde." Toxic Substances Portal Retrieved June 29, 2010, from www.atsdr.cdc.gov/substances/toxsubstance.asp?toxid=39.[2]

Alexandersson R, Hedenstierna G, Kolmodin-Hedman B. 1982. Exposure to formaldehyde: effects on pulmonary function. Arch Environ Health;37(5):279–84.

Alexandersson R, Hedenstierna G. 1989. Pulmonary function in wood workers exposed to formaldehyde: a prospective study. Arch Environ Health 44(1):5–11.

[ACGIH] American Conference of Governmental Industrial Hygienists. 1993. ACGIH announces change in formaldehyde TLV (threshold limit value). Health Hazard Mater Manage 6(6):6–7.

Anderson RC, Stock MF, Sawin R, Alarie Y. 1979. Toxicity of thermal decomposition products of urea formaldehyde and phenol formaldehyde foams. Toxicol App Pharmacol 51(1):9–17.

Baselt RC, Cravey RH. 1994. Disposition of toxic drugs and chemicals in man. 4th ed., Formaldehyde. 346–48.

Bender JR, Mullin LS, Graepel GJ, Wilson WE. 1983. Eye irritation response of humans to formaldehyde. AIHA J 44(6):463–5.

Bracken MJ, Leasa DJ, Morgan WK. 1985. Exposure to formaldehyde: relationship to respiratory symptoms and function. Can J Public Health 76(5):312–6.

Federal Register. 1992. Occupational exposure to formaldehyde—OSHA: Response to Court Remand; Final Rule. 102 Federal Register 22290–328.

Fischer, T., K. Andersen, et al. (1995). "Clinical standardization of the TRUE Test formaldehyde patch." Current Problems in Dermatology 22: 24-30.[2]

Garrett, M., M. Hooper, et al. (1999). "Increased Risk of Allergy in Children Due to Formaldehyde Exposure in Homes." Allergy 54: 330-337[2]

---

[2] CDC added this reference on December 15, 2010 in response to an Information Request for Correction http://aspe.hhs.gov/infoquality/request&response/35b8.pdf

Gordon SM, Callahan PJ, Nishioka MG, Brinkman MC, O'Rourke MK, Lebowitz MD. 1999. Residential environmental measurements in the national human exposure assessment survey (NHEXAS) pilot study in Arizona: preliminary results for pesticides and VOCs. J Exposure Anal Environ Epidemiol 9(5):456–470.

Hanrahan, L., M. Kay, et al. (1984). "Formaldehyde Vapor in Mobile Homes: A Cross Sectional Survey of Concentrations and Irritant Effects." American Journal of Public Health 74: 1026-1027[3]

Hendrick, D. and D. Lane (1977). "Occupational Formalin Asthma." British Journal of Industrial Medicine 34: 11-18. [3]

Hodgson AT, Rudd AF, Beal D, Chandra S. 2000. Volatile organic compound concentrations and emission rates in new manufactured and site-built houses. Indoor Air 10(3): 178–92.

Holness DL, Nethercott JR. 1989. Health status of funeral service workers exposed to formaldehyde. Arch Environ Health 44(4):222–8.

Horvath EP Jr, Anderson H Jr, Pierce WE, Hanrahan L, Wendlick JD. 1988. Effects of formaldehyde on the mucous membranes and lungs: a study of an industrial population. JAMA 259(5):701–7.

Imbus HR. 1985. Clinical evaluation of patients with complaints related to formaldehyde exposure. J Allergy Clin Immunol 76(6):831–40.

Institute of Medicine (2000). Clearing the Air: Asthma and Indoor Exposures. Washington DC, National Academy of Sciences. [3]

International Agency for Research on Cancer. 2004. Press Release N 153; June 15. Available from: http://www.iarc.fr/ENG/Press_Releases/archives/pr153a.html.

Jaakkola, J. J., H. Parise, et al. (2004). "Asthma, Wheezing, and Allergies in Russian Schoolchildren in Relation to New Surface Materials in the Home." American Journal of Public Health 94(4): 560-562.[3]

Kiec-Swierczynska, M. (1996). "Occupational allergic contact dermatitis in Lodz:1990-1994." Occup Med 48: 205-208. [3]

Kilburn KH, Warshaw R, Boylen CT, Johnson SJ, Seidman B, Sinclair R, et al. 1985. Pulmonary and neurobehavioral effects of formaldehyde exposure. Arch Environ Health 40(5):254–60.

---

[3] CDC added this reference on December 15, 2010 in response to an Information Request for Correction
http://aspe.hhs.gov/infoquality/request&response/35b8.pdf

Krzyzanowski, M., J. J. Quackenboss, et al. (1990). "Chronic respiratory effects of indoor formaldehyde exposure." Environmental Research 52(2): 117-125. [3]

Kulle TJ, Sauder LR, Hebel JR, Green DJ, Chatham MD. 1987. Formaldehyde dose-response in healthy nonsmokers. JAPCA 37(8):919–24.

Lee, H. K., Y. Alarie, et al. (1984). "Induction of formaldehyde sensitivity in guinea pigs." Toxicology and Applied Pharmacology 75(1): 147-155. [4]

Maibach, H. (1983). Formaldehyde: effects on animal and human skin. Formaldehyde Toxicity. J. Gibson. Washington DC, Hemisphere Publishing Corporation: 166-174. [4]

Main DM, Hogan TJ. 1983. Health effects of low-level exposure to formaldehyde. J Occup Med 25(12):896–900.

Malaka T, Kodama AM. 1990. Respiratory health of plywood workers occupationally exposed to formaldehyde. Arch Environ Health 45(5):288–94.

Marks, J., D. Belsito, et al. (1998). "North American Contact Dermatitis Group patch test results for the detection of delayed-type hypersensitivity of topical allergens." J Am Acad Dermatol 38: 911-918. [4]

McCoy, J. T. (2008). Formaldehyde. Spacecraft Maximum Allowable Concentrations for Selected Airborne Contaminants. C. o. T. Committee on Spacecraft Exposure Guidelines, National Research Council, National Academies Press. 5: 206-249. [4]

[NHLBI et al,.] National Heart, Lung, and Blood Institute, and National Asthma Education and Prevention Program Expert Panel (2007). Expert Panel Report 3:Guidelines for the Diagnosis and Management of Asthma. Bethesda, MD, US Department of Health and Human Services, National Institutes of Health. [4]

[NIOSH] National Institute for Occupational Safety and Health. 1992. Recommendations for Occupational Safety and Health: Compendium of Policy Documents and Statements. Available from: http://www.cdc.gov/niosh/92-100.html.

Nordman, H., H. Keskinen, et al. (1985). "Formaldehyde asthma -- Rare or overlooked?" J Allergy Clin Immunol 75: 91-99. [4]

Park JS, Ikeda K. 2006. Variations of formaldehyde and VOC levels during 3 years in new and older homes. Indoor Air (16):129–135

Ritchie IM, Lehnen RG. 1987. Formaldehyde-related health complaints of residents living in mobile and conventional homes. Am J Public Health 77(3):323–8.

---

[4] CDC added this reference on December 15, 2010 in response to an Information Request for Correction http://aspe.hhs.gov/infoquality/request&response/35b8.pdf

Rumchev, K., J. Spickett, et al. (2002). "Domestic Exposure to Formaldehyde Significantly Increases the Risk of Asthma in Young Children." European Respiratory Journal 20(403-408).[5]

Staab, C., M. Hellgren, et al. (2008). "Dual Functions of Alcohol dehydrogenase 3: implications with focus on formaldehyde and S-nitrosolglutathione reductase activities." Cellular and Molecular Life Sciences 65: 3950-3960. [5]

Stock TH, Mendez SR. 1985. A survey of typical exposures to formaldehyde in Houston area residences. AIHA J 46(6):313–7.

Sullivan JB, Krieger GR. 2001. Clinical environmental health and toxic exposures. 2nd ed. Formaldehyde 1006–14.

Thompson, C. M. and R. C. Grafstrom (2008). "Mechanistic Considerations for Formaldehyde-Induced Bronchoconstriction Involving S-Nitroglutathione Reductase." Journal of Toxicology and Environmental Health Part A 71: 244-248. [5]

[US CPSC] US Consumer Product Safety Commission 1982. Release # 82-005. Available from: http://classaction.findlaw.com/recall/cpsc/files/1982mar/82005.html.

[US CPSC] US Consumer Product Safety Commission. 1997. An update on formaldehyde. 1997 Revision. Available from: http://www.cpsc.gov/cpscpub/pubs/725.pdf.

US Department of Labor. Occupational Exposure to Formaldehyde. 2007. http://www.pp.okstate.edu/ehs/training/OSHAFHYD.HTM.

[US EPA] US Environmental Protection Agency. 2007. Indoor Air Quality—Formaldehyde. Retrieved from http://www.epa.gov/iaq/pubs/insidest.html#Look6 on January 15th, 2008.

Wantke, F. and Wantke (1996). "Exposure to gaseous formaldehyde induces IgE-mediated sensitization to formaldehyde in school-children." Clinical and experimental allergy 26(3): 276. [5]

Weisel CP, Zhang J, Turpin BJ, Morandi MT, Colome S, Stock TH, et al. 2005. Relationships of indoor, outdoor, and personal air (RIOPA). Part I. Collection methods and descriptive analyses. Research Report (Health Effects Institute) (130 Pt 1):1–107; discussion 109–27.

[WHO] World Health Organization. 1989. Environmental health criteria for formaldehyde. Geneva, Switzerland: World Health Organization; Volume 89.

---

[5] CDC added this reference on December 15, 2010 in response to an Information Request for Correction
http://aspe hhs.gov/infoquality/request&response/35b8.pdf

Figure 1. Recruitment of Participants in a Study of Occupied FEMA-Supplied Trailers in Louisiana and Mississippi, December 2007–January 2008

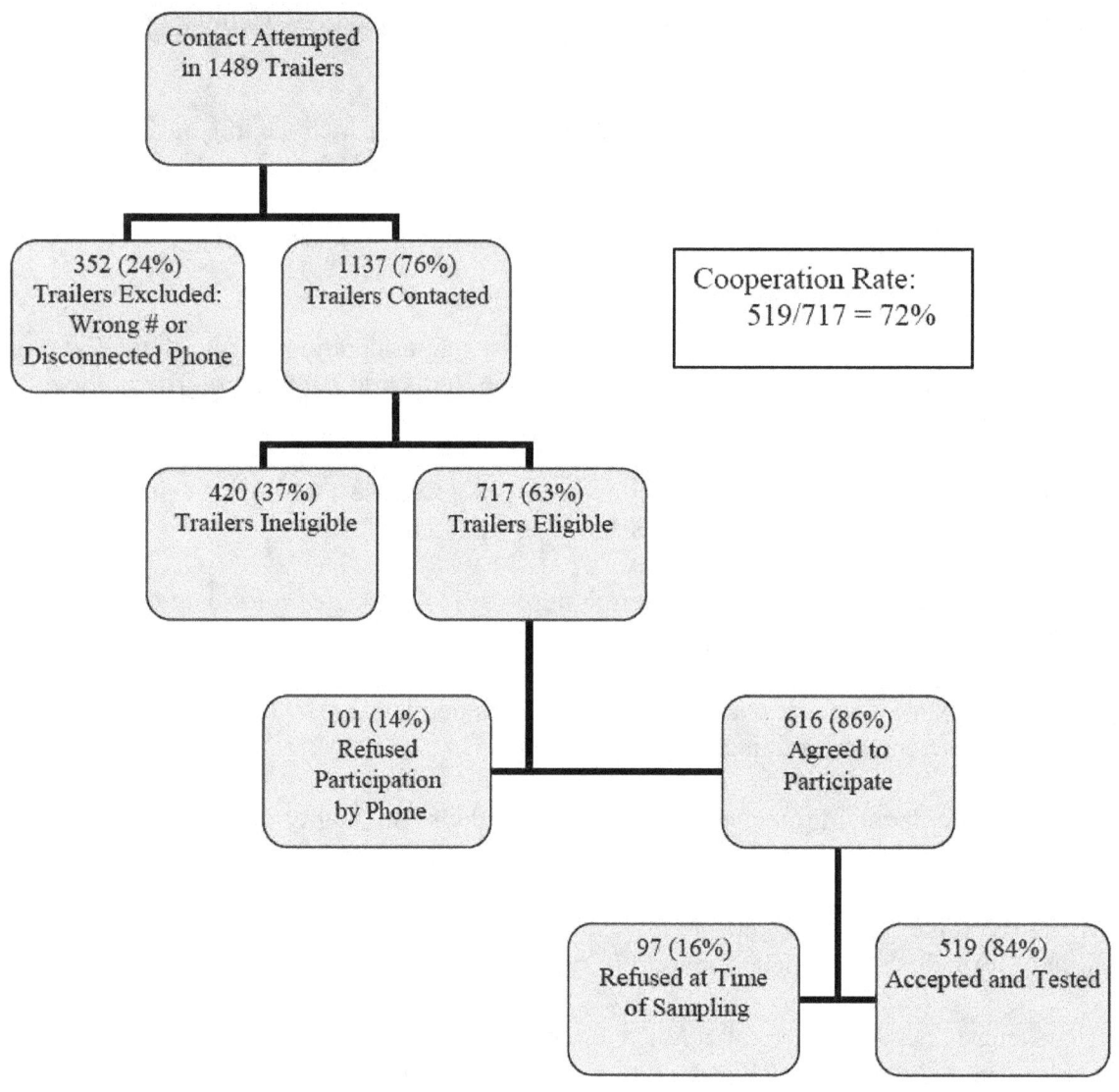

Figure 2. Geometric Mean Formaldehyde Levels in Occupied FEMA-Supplied Trailers, Louisiana and Mississippi, December 2007–January 2008

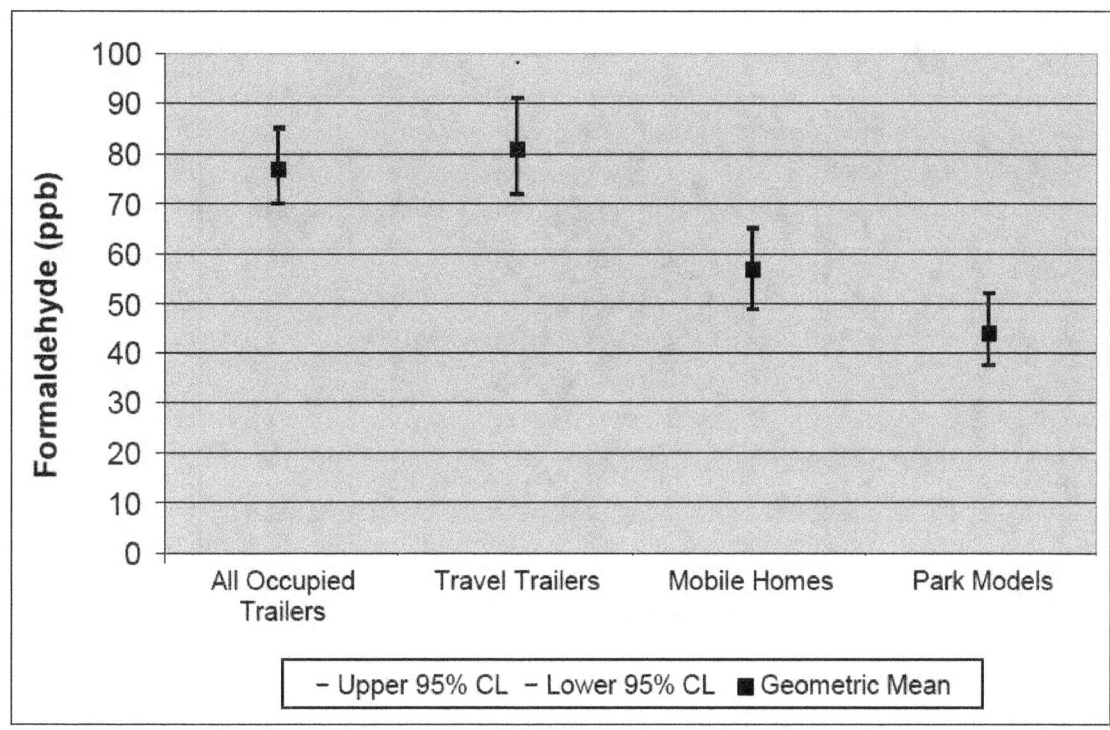

GM = geometric mean; ppb = parts per billion (divide by 1000 to get parts per million); CL = confidence limit.

Figure 3. Association of Indoor Temperature with Natural Log Formaldehyde Levels in Occupied FEMA-supplied Trailers in Louisiana and Mississippi, December 2007– January 2008

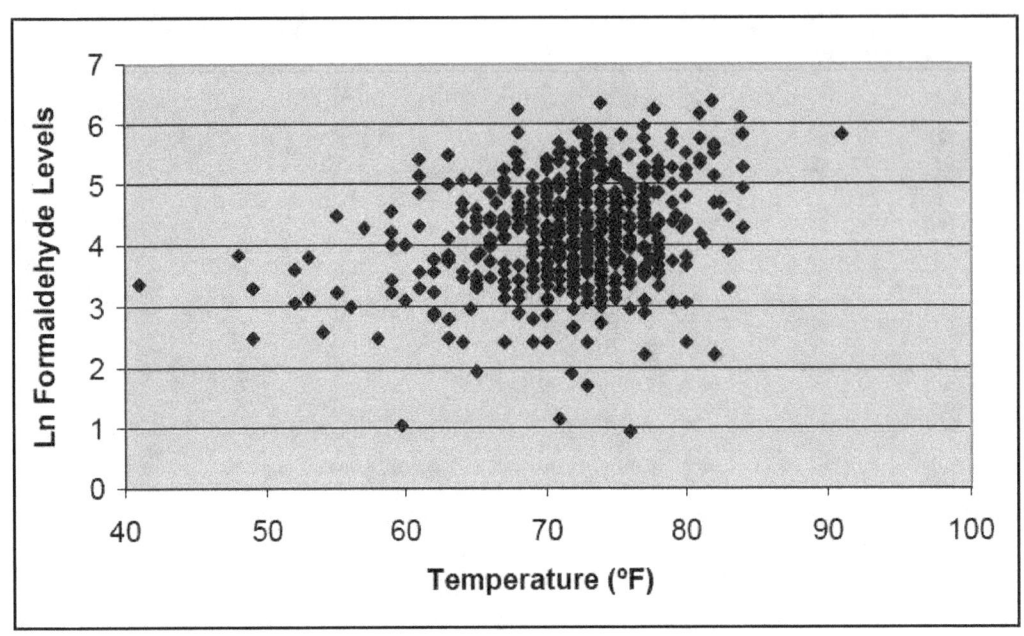

Range: 41°F–91°F

Figure 4. Association of Indoor Relative Humidity with Natural Log Formaldehyde Levels in Occupied FEMA-supplied Trailers in Louisiana and Mississippi, December 2007–January 2008

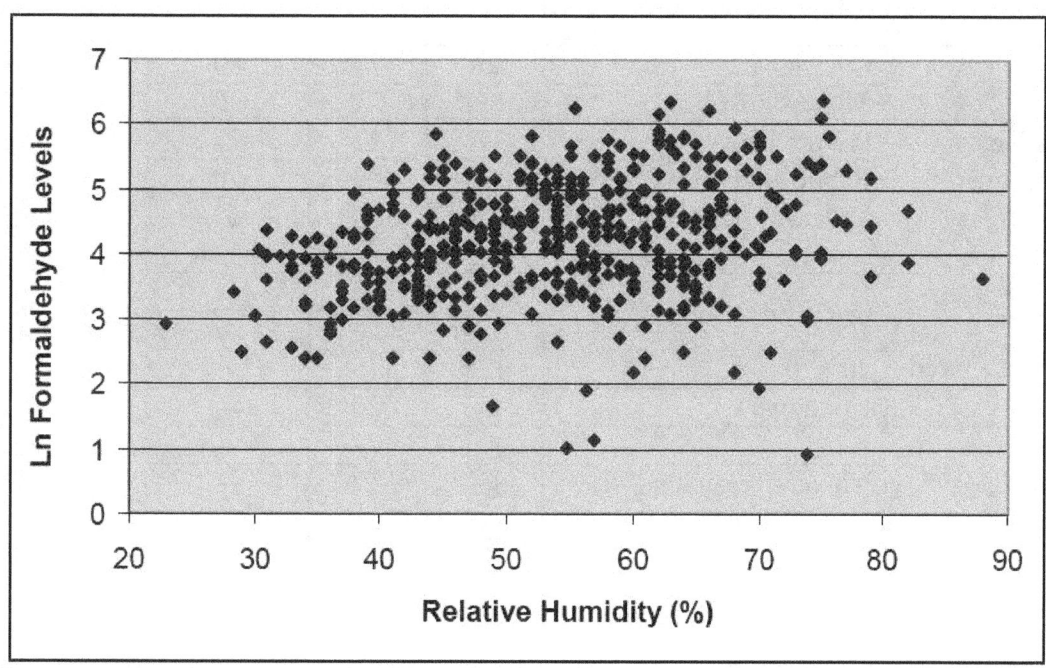

Range: 23%–88% relative humidity.

Table 1. Demographics of Trailers and Occupants in 519 Occupied FEMA-Supplied Trailers in Louisiana and Mississippi, December 2007–January 2008

Category	Variable	No.	(%)	Weighted (%)
State	Louisiana	408	79	80
	Mississippi	111	21	20
Trailer locations	Private land	374	72	77
	Public land	127	24	20
	Unknown/Undetermined	18	3	3
Year trailer was manufactured				
	2005	258	50	--
	2006	128	25	--
	Unknown	133	26	--
Residents			--	--
	No. adult residents (age ≥ 18 years)	852	77	--
	No. teen residents (age $13 \leq 17$ years)	97	9	--
	No. child residents (age $3 \leq 12$ years)	120	11	--
	No. baby residents (age ≤ 2 years)	41	4	--
	Average no. residents per trailer	2	--	--
Utilities	Paid by occupant	420	81	83
	Paid by FEMA	90	17	16
	Paid by other	9	2	1

Table 2. Formaldehyde Levels in 519 Occupied FEMA-Supplied Trailers in Louisiana and Mississippi, December 2007–January 2008

Trailer Type	No.	Formaldehyde GM (ppb)	Range (ppb)	95% CI for GM (ppb)	Weighted Percentage of the Sample with Levels	
					≥ 100 ppb	≥ 300 ppb
Travel trailer	360	81	3–590	72–92	42%	5%
Park model	90	44	3–170	38–53	14%	0%
Mobile home	69	57	11–320	49–65	9%	<1%

GM = Geometric mean; ppb = parts per billion (divide by 1000 to get parts per million); CI = confidence interval.

Final CDC Findings—Formaldehyde Levels in FEMA-Supplied Trailers

Table 3. Formaldehyde Levels by Manufacturer in 519 Occupied FEMA-Supplied Trailers in Louisiana and Mississippi, December 2007–January 2008

Home Type	Brand	No. in stratum	No. in sample	Formaldehyde GM (ppb)	Range (ppb)	95% CI for GM (ppb)	Weighted Percentage of the Sample with Levels	
							≥100 ppb	≥300 ppb
Travel trailer	Gulfstream	14,624	123	104	3–590	88–123	56%	9%
	Forest River	3,220	36	82	17–510	61–109	42%	6%
	Fleetwood	2,371	47	39	3–140	32–48	6%	0%
	Fleetwood CA	1,699	39	43	7–300	34–55	13%	3%
	Pilgrim	1,584	39	108	25–520	85–136	51%	3%
	Keystone	1,395	38	102	23–480	79–131	53%	11%
	Other	15,637	38	74	11–330	57–96	37%	3%
Park model	Silver Creek	224	53	33	3–170	29–39	6%	0%
	Other	809	37	48	11–160	39–60	16%	0%
Mobile home	Cavalier	921	42	78	14–320	65–95	36%	2%
	Other	4,486	27	53	11–120	45–63	4%	0%
	Total	46,970	519	77	3–590	70–85	38%	5%

GM = geometric mean; ppb = parts per billion (divide by 1000 to get parts per million); CI = confidence interval.

Table 4. Activities Reported by Occupants in 519 Occupied FEMA-Supplied Trailers in Louisiana and Mississippi, December 2007–January 2008

Category	Variable	No.	(%)	Weighted (%)
Temperature and ventilation	No. hours air conditioning used per day in week before testing			
	<1 hour	212	41	44
	1–4 hours	136	26	27
	5–8 hours	56	11	10
	>8 hours	82	16	13
	Don't know	33	6	6
	No. hours heat used per day in 2 weeks before testing			
	<1 hour	134	26	28
	1–4 hours	154	30	29
	5–8 hours	98	19	21
	>8 hours	106	20	16
	Don't know	27	5	6
	Space heaters regularly used			
	Yes	198	38	44
	No	301	58	53
	Don't know	20	4	2
	Windows/doors/scuttles left open within 3 hours before testing			
	Yes	202	39	44
	No	299	58	54
	Don't know	18	3	2
	Time windows/doors/scuttles left open before testing			
	<1 hour	171	33	37
	1–4 hours	75	14	14
	5–8 hours	9	2	2
	>8 hours	41	8	10
	Don't know	223	43	37
Smoking	No. people who have smoked in trailer the prior 2 weeks			
	None	335	65	66
	1	112	22	21
	≥2	72	14	13
	Someone smoked in the 3 hours before testing			
	Yes	105	20	19
	No	399	77	79
	Don't know	15	3	2
Cooking	Anyone cook in trailer			

	Yes	410	79	81
	No	82	16	15
	Don't know	27	5	4
	Anyone cook in trailer in the 3 hours before testing:			
	Yes	86	17	14
	No	397	76	80
	Don't know	11	2	2
	Question skipped	25	5	5
Time indoors	Average amount of time per day respondent spent inside trailer			
	<1 hour	0	0	0
	1–4 hours	9	2	1
	5–8 hours	70	13	14
	>8 hours	424	82	82
	Don't know	16	3	3
	Household member sleeps in trailer			
	Yes	482	93	93
	No	13	3	3
	Don't know	24	5	4
Pets	No. trailers with at least 1 dog	113	22	20
	No. trailers with at least 1 cat	30	6	5
	No. trailers with at least 1 bird	10	2	1
	No. trailers with other pets	11	2	1
Products used	Pesticides sprayed in past month:			
	Yes	86	17	17
	No	410	79	79
	Don't know	23	4	4
	Candles used in the week before testing			
	Yes	128	25	24
	No	391	75	76
	Air freshener used in week before testing			
	Yes	308	59	61
	No	211	41	39
	Glue, paint, or furniture finish used in week before testing			
	Yes	17	3	3
	No	502	97	97
	Mothballs used in week before testing			
	Yes	5	1	1
	No	514	99	99

	Closet Fresh used in week before testing			
	Yes	5	1	1
	No	514	99	99
	Nail polish used in week before testing			
	Yes	53	10	9
	No	466	90	91
Trailer condition	Roof leaked in the past 3 months			
	Yes	72	14	17
	No	412	79	77
	Don't know	35	7	6
	Pipe leaked in past 3 months			
	Yes	70	13	15
	No	427	82	81
	Don't know	22	4	4
	Reported mold in past 3 months			
	Yes	93	18	21
	No	403	78	75
	Don't know	23	4	3

Table 5. Walk-Through Observations by Investigators in 519 Occupied FEMA-Supplied Trailers in Louisiana and Mississippi, December 2007–January 2008

Category	Variable	No.	(%)	Weighted (%)
Trailer characteristics	Problems seen with the roof			
	Yes	33	6	6
	No	483	93	93
	Don't know	3	1	<1
	Signs that water spills onto siding			
	Yes	66	13	13
	No	453	87	87
	Signs of mold in living area of trailer			
	Yes, <1 ft^2	26	5	4
	Yes, 1–4 ft^2	17	3	4
	Yes, >4 ft^2	11	2	2
	No	465	90	90
	Carpeting in trailer			
	Yes	191	37	43
	No	328	63	57
Air conditioning	Forced air			
	Yes	273	53	40
	No	246	47	60
	Rooftop air conditioning			
	Yes	224	43	57
	No	295	57	43
	No working air conditioning			
	Yes	3	1	<1
	No	516	99	99
	Other type of air conditioning			
	Yes	7	1	<1
	No	512	99	99
Heating	Central heating/forced air			
	Yes	463	89	89
	No	56	11	11
	Space heater			
	Yes	91	18	21
	No	428	82	79
	No working heating system			
	Yes	2	<1	1
	No	517	99	99
	Other type of heating system			
	Yes	16	3	2
	No	503	97	98

Fuel source for cooking	Electricity			
	Yes	214	41	23
	No	305	59	77
	Propane gas			
	Yes	272	52	71
	No	247	48	29
	Natural gas			
	Yes	3	1	<1
	No	516	99	99
	Charcoal or wood			
	Yes	0	0	0
	No	519	100	100
	Other			
	Yes	7	1	2
	No	512	99	98
Smoke detectors	Functioning smoke detectors			
	Yes	390	75	71
	No	129	25	29

Table 6. Adjusted Geometric Mean Formaldehyde Level from Occupied FEMA-Supplied Trailers in Louisiana and Mississippi that Had Mold (≥ 1 ft^2), December 2007–January 2008, from Multivariate Analysis

Mold ≥ 1 ft^2	No. Trailers	Adjusted GM Formaldehyde (ppb)*
Yes	28	86
No	491	63

*Adjusted for stratum, average temperature, relative humidity, and open windows/doors/scuttles 3 hours before testing (all significant multivariate variables). GM=geometric mean.

Table 7. Adjusted Geometric Mean Formaldehyde Level from Occupied FEMA-Supplied Trailers in Louisiana and Mississippi that Had Open Windows, Doors, or Scuttles 3 Hours Before Testing, December 2007–January 2008, from Multivariate Model

Windows/Doors/ Scuttles Open	No. Trailers	Adjusted GM Formaldehyde (ppb)*
Yes	202	65
No	299	83

*Adjusted for stratum, average temperature, relative humidity, and presence of mold (≥ 1 ft^2) (all significant multivariate variables). GM=geometric mean.

Table 8. Adjusted Geometric Mean Formaldehyde Level from Occupied FEMA-Supplied Trailers in Louisiana and Mississippi, by Stratum, December 2007–January 2008, from Multivariate Model

Stratum	Adjusted GM Formaldehyde Level (ppb)*
Travel trailer	
Gulfstream	111
Pilgrim	129
Fleetwood CA	44
Fleetwood	42
Forest River	102
Keystone	122
Other	90
Park model	
Silver Creek	37
Other	55
Mobile home	
Cavalier	84
Other	62

*Adjusted for average temperature, relative humidity, windows/doors/scuttles open 3 hours before testing, and presence of mold (≥ 1 ft^2) (all significant multivariate variables). GM = geometric mean.

Table 9. Estimated Regression Coefficients for Modeling of Statistically Significant Variables of Occupied FEMA-Supplied Trailers in Louisiana and Mississippi, December 2007–January 2008

Variable	Estimate	*P* value
Intercept	0.012 (α)	0.983
Gulfstream travel trailer	Reference group	
Pilgrim	0.148 (β_1)	0.232
Fleetwood CA	- 0.917 (β_2)	<0.001
Fleetwood	- 0.965 (β_3)	<0.001
Forest River	- 0.085 (β_4)	0.600
Keystone	0.096 (β_5)	0.477
Other travel trailer	- 0.215 (β_6)	0.114
Silver Creek park model	- 1.094 (β_7)	<0.001
Other park model	- 0.695 (β_8)	<0.001
Cavalier mobile home	-0.275 (β_9)	0.016
Other mobile home	- 0.583 (β_{10})	<0.001
Temperature (°F)	0.052 (β_{11})	<0.001
Relative humidity (%)	0.017 (β_{12})	<0.001
Windows/doors/scuttles open (yes)	- 0.243 (β_{13})	0.017
Mold (≥ 1 ft^2)	0.311 (β_{14})	0.052

y = natural log of formaldehyde levels (ppb).

Formaldehyde Level Multivariate Model:

$y = 0.012 + 0.148x_1 - 0.917x_2 - 0.965x_3 - 0.085x_4 + 0.096x_5 - 0.215x_6 - 1.094x_7 - 0.695x_8$

$- 0.275x_9 - 0.583x_{10} + 0.052x_{11} + 0.017x_{12} - 0.243x_{13} + 0.311x_{14}$

APPENDIX A:
PROTOCOL FOR TRAILER SELECTION AND RECRUITMENT

CONTACTING PARTICIPANTS: Materials needed
1. You will receive a stratified list of names and up to 3 phone numbers of residents in trailers from a CDC representative. This list represents the people whom you will contact for participation in the study.
2. For each trailer, you will need one clean phone log form (Appendix B) to log all attempted and successful calls.
3. You will need a copy of the telephone script (Appendix B) to ensure that each conversation is consistent.
4. You will need a clean copy of the "Obtaining Assent" form (Appendix C) for each trailer contacted.

CONTACTING PARTICIPANTS: Conducting the phone calls
1. You will need to make the calls from the provided spreadsheet.
2. Begin with the first name on the list and call them using the first number provided.
3. If you are unable to get an answer, try the next phone number provided.
4. After each attempt, record the information in the phone log (Appendix B).
5. **Fifteen attempts** using each provided number must be made before ending the recruitment of the person from the contact list. **Over half** of these attempts should be made after 5 pm in the event that the contacts are not at home to receive the call during the day.

   If you are unable to reach a contact:
6. If you are unable to contact a trailer after making fifteen attempts for each provided phone number, the majority of which attempted after 5 pm, file the recorded phone log into a folder labeled "Unable to Contact".

   If you are able to contact a person in the trailer:
7. When someone answers the phone, use the phone script (Appendix B) to guide the conversation.
8. If the adult resident is not available, you will need to continue efforts to make contact with him/her.
9. If the adult resident is NOT interested in participating, note refusal in the phone log. File the phone log into a folder labeled "Refused".
10. If the adult resident is interested in participating, ensure that they are eligible using the criteria outlined in the phone script.
11. If the adult resident agrees to participate, obtain verbal assent (Appendix C) and set up an appointment date and time with the adult resident.
12. Record "Agreed" in the phone log and file the phone log AND assent form in a folder labeled "Agreed".

RECRUITMENT COMPLETION
1. Recruitment is complete when all 11 strata have been completed. This will consist of at least 500 trailers total.

PARTICIPANT FOLLOW-UP: Appointment reminder
1. Prior to their appointment, call the adult resident to confirm the sampling date and time
2. If the respondent can no longer make the appointment, reschedule the appointment.

APPENDIX B:
PHONE LOG FOR PARTICIPANT RECRUITMENT

Interviewer initials   _____

Number on spreadsheet   _____

Trailer VIN   _____

Address   _____

Adult resident name   _____

Phone number (s)   1:_____

                               2:_____

                               3:_____

Interviewer must make at least **15 attempts for each provided phone number** (of which, **half** of the attempts must be conducted in the evening, after 5 pm) to contact each potential trailer.

Date called (mm/dd/yy)	Time called (am/pm)	Phone number called (1, 2, or 3)	I=For initial contact F=Follow-up call A=Name of alternative adult resident representative	Status (No answer, Left message, Call back, Agreed, Refused, Excluded)	Recommended call back time (am/pm)

APPENDIX B, con't:
TELEPHONE SCRIPT FOR PARTICIPANT RECRUITMENT

IF CHILD ANSWERS THE PHONE:

Hi, may I speak with your mother or father please?

> IF NO ADULT IS HOME:
>
> Okay. Could you please tell me what would be a good time to call back?
>
> *[NOTE IN PHONE LOG]*
>
> Thank you, I'll try calling back later.

IF AN ADULT ANSWERS THE PHONE:

Hello, this is _____ calling for the Centers for Disease Control and Prevention. Is this the _____(NAME)_____residence? I am working with FEMA and the Louisiana and Mississippi Departments of Public Health to find out if there is formaldehyde (a potentially harmful chemical) in the trailers in which people are living. We have picked some trailers at random, like flipping a coin. May I ask if you are an adult resident living in a FEMA-owned trailer?

> IF NO,
>
>> Okay, we will be working with all adult residents who are 18 years or older. What is a good time to call back to speak with him or her? And is this the best number to reach him/her?
>>
>> *[NOTE NAME AND TIME IN PHONE LOG]*
>>
>> Thank you, I'll try calling back later.

> IF YES,
>
>> We are asking the people who live in the trailers to let us test the indoor air for formaldehyde. We have picked your trailer as one that we would like to test.
>> What we learn will help the federal government make decisions about if some people need to be moved out of their trailers to protect their health. For your inconvenience, a $50 gift card will be given to you at the completion of the study. Participation is voluntary. Do you think you may be interested in participating?
>>
>>> *IF NO*
>>> Thank you. I appreciate you taking time out to talk.
>>>
>>> *IF YES*

Great. I would like to first ask you a few questions about yourself and your trailer. GO TO CRITERIA (below)

CRITERIA

1. Are you, as an adult resident, 18 years in age or older?
   - ☐ If YES, continue to question 2
   - ☐ If NO, go to "End of interview for exclusions"

2. Do you still live in a FEMA-issued trailer more than 6 hours per day?
   - ☐ If YES, continue to next section
   - ☐ If NO, go to "End of interview for exclusions"

IF YES is answered for questions 1-2:

If you agree to have us test your trailer, several things will take place:

1. We will set up a time to visit your trailer soon. The visit will not take more than an hour and a half. Cooking and smoking will not be allowed during the testing process.
2. We will ask you some questions about how you cook in your home and if people smoke in your home.
3. We will look around your home and fill out a short form about what type of heating you have, what type of stove you cook on, what type of air conditioner you have, and other similar questions.
4. We will test your trailer for formaldehyde and will also measure the temperature and humidity. We will deliver the test results of your trailer to you about a month after we test it.
5. For your time and inconvenience, you will also receive a $50 gift card

Are you interested in participating in this study?

IF YES
   GO TO "WHEN SOMEONE AGREES TO PARTICIPATE"

IF NO
   Okay, thank you so much for your time.
   [HANG UP AND RECORD IN PHONE LOG AS REFUSAL]

END OF INTERVIEW FOR EXCLUSIONS

Thank you very much for your interest and for your willingness to be in the study. Unfortunately, it is important that people in our study be the adult resident and are 18 years or older. Also, because we are interested in the formaldehyde levels that people are currently exposed to, we are working with those who are still living in their FEMA-issued trailer. Thank you again for your time. *[RECORD AS EXCLUSION IN PHONE LOG]*

WHEN SOMEONE AGREES TO PARTICIPATE
Go to Appendix C: OBTAINING ASSENT *[RECORD AS AGREED IN PHONE LOG]*

APPENDIX C:
OBTAINING ASSENT

Thank you for helping us with this important project. Everything you tell us and all your test results will be kept private to the extent allowed by the law. To protect your privacy, we will not put your name on the project forms, but we will write down your trailer's address or a unique identification number assigned by the CDC.

You can change your mind and decide that you do not want us to test your trailer. If you do change your mind, it will not affect any of your benefits from the Federal Government.

_____   _____   _____
Adult resident's Name   Date   Time

_____   _____   _____
Person Obtaining Assent   Date   Time

_____

"In my opinion, this person cannot give informed assent."

_____   _____   _____
Person conducting telephone interview   Date   Time

APPENDIX D:
INFORMED CONSENT FOR PARTICIPATION

Evaluation of Formaldehyde in Occupied FEMA Owned Temporary Housing Units

> For all potential participants, the informed consent document will be available for the participant to read or, if requested by the participant, will be read out loud. Participants will be required to provide a signature to document informed consent. The informed consent document will request permission for collection and testing of a laboratory sample.

(Flesch-Kincaid Reading Level for English text below = 5.2)

1. Introduction and purpose

We are working for the Centers for Disease Control and Prevention (CDC). CDC is working with the Federal Emergency Management Agency (FEMA) to find out whether there is formaldehyde (a potentially harmful chemical) in the trailers people are living in. We have picked some trailers at random, like flipping a coin. We are asking the people who live in those trailers to let us test their inside air for formaldehyde. We have picked your trailer as one that we would like to test. What we learn will help CDC and FEMA make decisions on housing placement priorities and if some people need to be moved into different trailers to protect their health. The testing process will include air testing which will take no more than one hour and a half. At the same time there will be a brief inspection of the trailer for up to 30 minutes, and some questions to be answered by you for up to 15 minutes. Section 301 of the Public Health Act permits us to collect such information. No cooking or smoking will be allowed during the testing process.

We are doing this testing in a scientifically valid way. That means that we choose the trailers to test instead of letting people ask to have their trailer tested. You and FEMA will learn the formaldehyde level in your trailer, and FEMA will learn the formaldehyde levels across many other trailers. This will help FEMA make decisions to protect people's health.

2. Freedom of choice

You can choose to be part of this project or not. We will explain what we want to do to you so you can decide. Please ask us questions if you do not understand something. If you choose to be part of this project, you will need to sign this form. Then we will give you a copy of this form.

3. Benefits/Risks

If you agree to be in this evaluation, you can learn more about your home environment. If the formaldehyde level in your trailer is high, you may be given priority for housing relocation.

4. Confidentiality

Everything you tell us and all your test results will be kept private to the extent allowed by the law. To protect your privacy, we will not put your name on the project forms, but we will write down your trailer's address or a unique identification number assigned by the CDC. We will tell FEMA about the levels of formaldehyde in each trailer. Personally identifying data will be destroyed by the CDC, but left at the Louisiana and Mississippi Departments of Public Health at the completion of the study.

5. Cost/Payment

It will not cost you anything to have your trailer tested as part of this project. You will be compensated for your time and inconvenience with a $50 gift card at the completion of the study.

6. Right to refuse or withdraw

Before we start, we want to make sure you understand that it is up to you whether or not to join this project. You have the right to ask us to stop the testing at any time for any reason.

7. Persons to contact

If you have any questions please feel free to ask us now.

If you have questions later, please contact:
Matt Murphy at 770-488-3417 or
Gary Noonan at 770-488-3449

If you feel that you have been harmed by this evaluation or if you have any concerns about your rights, please contact the CDC Deputy Associate Director for Science in Atlanta, Georgia, USA at 800-584-8814.

8. Your consent

I agree to allow the air in my trailer to be tested. The information in this informed consent form has been explained to me. I have been given a chance to ask questions. I feel that all of my questions have been answered. I know that it is my choice to allow the air testing or not. I know that if I agree to the testing I can have it stopped at any time.

I give permission for an air sample to be collected and tested for formaldehyde, and for the temperature and humidity to be measured in my home.	□ YES	□ NO

I have read or had this form read to me. By signing below, I consent to the air testing and to providing answers to the survey questions.

_____   _____
Name and signature of participant   Date (mm/dd/yyyy)

_____ _____
Name and signature of witness   Date (mm/dd/yyyy)

| Office use only |
| Place ID label here |

APPENDIX E:
EXPOSURE ASSESSMENT QUESTIONNAIRE AND WALK THROUGH
SURVEY

INTERVIEWER SCRIPT:

The purpose of this part of the interview is to collect some information about you and your FEMA trailer environment. If there is a question that you do not want to answer, please let me know and we can skip it. All of your responses will be kept private and will not affect any of the home or health care services that you currently receive.

This interview will begin with a few questions about your age and where you work. We will then look at the inside and outside of your trailer. We will walk around and through your trailer with you to make some observations.

Form Approved

OMB No. 0920-0008

Expiration Date 3/31/2010

EXPOSURE ASSESSMENT QUESTIONNAIRE AND
WALK THROUGH SURVEY

Date _____ (mm/dd/yyyy)
Interviewer initials _____

Trailer VIN _____   Trailer barcode _____
Trailer type: ☐ Travel trailer   ☐ Mobile home   ☐ Park   ☐ Other

Street address:
_____
County: _____   State (circle one): LA / MS
Zip code: _____

Is this home located on private land or in a federal/commercially owned park?
☐ Private land   ☐ Park
If a park, please indicate the park name: _____

Trailer occupied since _____ (mm/dd/yyyy)

Who pays for your utilities?   ☐ Self   ☐ FEMA   ☐ Other

Total number of residents in trailer   _____

Number of residents in trailer, by age group _____ adults   (≥18 years)
                                              _____ children (≥13-<18 yrs)
                                              _____ children (3-<13 yrs)
                                              _____ children (<3 yrs)

May we contact you if we have any additional questions?   ☐ Yes   ☐ No
If YES, what is the best phone number to use and time of day to call?

Phone: (   ) _____   Time: _____ AM / PM
Alternate: (   ) _____   Time: _____ AM / PM

suggestions for reducing this burden to CDC/ATSDR Reports Clearance Officer; 1600 Clifton Road NE, MS D-74, Atlanta, Georgia 30333; ATTN: PRA (0920-0008)

INTERVIEWER QUESTIONNAIRE

Pests		
1.	Have pesticides been sprayed inside your home the past **month**?	❑ Yes ❑ No ❑ Don't know
Indoor environment		
2.	Does your trailer have air conditioning?	❑ Yes ❑ No **(go to question # 4)**
3.	During the **past 2 weeks**, how many hours—on average—did you keep your air conditioning running every day?	❑ Less than 1 hour ❑ 1–4 hours ❑ 5–8 hours ❑ More than 8 hours ❑ Don't know
4.	During the **past 2 weeks**, how many hours—on average—did you keep your heater running every day?	❑ Less than 1 hour ❑ 1–4 hours ❑ 5–8 hours ❑ More than 8 hours ❑ Don't know ❑ No working heater in trailer
5.	Do you regularly use space heaters?	❑ Yes ❑ No ❑ Don't know
6.	Were the windows, scuttles, and/or door open in the past 3 hours?	❑ Yes ❑ No **(go to question # 8)** ❑ Don't know
7.	Approximately how long did you keep your windows and/or door open **before this visit**?	❑ Less than 1 hour ❑ 1–4 hours ❑ 5–8 hours ❑ More than 8 hours ❑ Don't know
8.	Did anyone smoke in here in the past 3 hours?	❑ Yes ❑ No ❑ Don't know
9.	During the past **two weeks**, how many people have smoked in here?	# People:_____
10.	How many packs of cigarettes are smoked in this house each day?	❑ None ❑ < ½ pack ❑ ½ - 1 pack ❑ >1 – 2 packs ❑ > 2 packs ❑ Don't know
11.	Does anyone cook in here?	❑ Yes ❑ No **(go to question #13)**

		❑ Don't know
12.	Did anyone cook in here the past 3 hours?	❑ Yes ❑ No ❑ Don't know

Daily activities

13.	What is the average amount of time that you spend inside your trailer each day?	❑ Less than one hour ❑ 1-4 hours ❑ 5-8 hours ❑ More than 8 hours ❑ Don't know
14.	Do you or your household members sleep in this trailer?	❑ Yes ❑ No ❑ Don't know
15.	Were any of the following used here in the past week?	❑ Candles ❑ Air fresheners ❑ Glue, paint, furniture finish ❑ Mothballs ❑ Closet fresh (mildewcide) ❑ Nail polish
16.	Do you have any pets that you keep in here and how many?	❑ Dog #:_____ ❑ Cat #:_____ ❑ Bird #:_____ ❑ Other: #:
17.	Have you noticed the roof leaking in the past 3 months?	❑ Yes ❑ No ❑ Don't know
18.	Have you noticed pipes leaking in the past 3 months?	❑ Yes ❑ No ❑ Don't know
19.	Have you noticed mold in your home during the past 3 months?	❑ Yes ❑ No ❑ Don't know

Questions pertaining to the trailer		(Check all that apply)
1.	Do you see any problems with the roof (for example sagging or holes)?	❑ Yes ❑ No ❑ Unable to see entire roof
2.	Are there signs that water spills onto siding?	❑ Yes ❑ No
3.	Are there any signs of mold in the living area of the trailer?	❑ Yes ❑ No If **YES**, estimate size of mold growth? ❑ < 1 sq. foot ❑ 1-4 sq. feet ❑ > 4 sq. feet
4.	Is there carpeting in the trailer?	❑ Yes ❑ No
5.	What type of air conditioning does the trailer have?	❑ Central AC/forced air ❑ AC/chiller on roof of Trailer ❑ No working AC system ❑ Other: _____
6.	What type of heating does the trailer have?	❑ Central heating/forced air ❑ Space heaters ❑ No working heating system ❑ Other: _____
7.	What type fuels are used for cooking?	❑ Electricity ❑ Propane Gas ❑ Natural Gas ❑ Charcoal or wood ❑ Other:_____
8.	Is there a functioning smoke detector?	❑ Yes ❑ No

Notes: _____

_____

APPENDIX F:

ENVIRONMENTAL SAMPLING PROTOCOL

Formaldehyde Samples

Analysis Method:

Formaldehyde samples will be collected using the NIOSH Manual of Analytical Methods (NMAM) Method 2016 with Supelco S10 LpDNPH cartridges. The limit of detection (LOD) shall be 0.07 microgram per sample and the limit of quantification (LOQ) shall be 0.23 microgram. Lower LOD and LOQ are acceptable. A minimum quantifiable concentration of 0.0063 parts per million is required with a 30 liter sample volume collected over one hour. The definition from the NMAM should be used for LOD and LOQ (http://www.cdc.gov/niosh/nmam/pdfs/glossary.pdf).

Sample Collection:

Samples will be collected at a flow rate of 500 ± 50 milliliters per minute for one hour. Each sample will be collected in the center of the trailer primary living room on a four foot tall stand that mimics the breathing zone height of an adult when sitting. Residents will be asked to configure doors and windows as they would have them while they slept. Sampling will be under observation by one of the sampling team members at all times. Every tenth sample collected by a team will be a duplicate sample. Sampling will occur during a specific window of time per day for all trailers which is between 10:00 AM – 8:00 PM. No cooking or smoking in the trailer will be allowed during the one-hour sample collection period.

Quality Assurance and Control:

Six to ten, or additional as required by the lab, <u>media blanks</u> will be taken from each lot of sample tubes. The media blanks should be taken from the start of a lot (2 to 3), from the middle of a lot (2 to 4) and from the end of a lot (2 to 3). All media blanks should be logged on the chain of custody sheet and sent for analysis on the day that they were collected with the field blanks and samples.

Two to ten, or additional as required by the lab, <u>field blanks</u> will be collected on each day in which samples are collected. This can be divided by travel groups, (groups consisting of teams that are operating in close proximity or who are traveling together). All field blanks should be logged on the chain of custody sheet and sent for analysis on the day that they were collected with the media blanks and samples.

Sample Handling:

Sample tubes will be stored in a freezer or in a cooler on ice at all times (upon receipt, while not being used for sampling, and during shipment to the laboratory).

At the end of each sampling day samples will be shipped to the analytical laboratory either overnight or if collected after the last overnight drop off time the next morning in coolers with chain of custody documents enclosed or attached. Samples collected on Saturday and Sunday will be stored on ice or in a freezer and shipped by overnight means with the appropriate chain of custody documents to the analytical laboratory on the following Monday morning.

Temperature and Relative Humidity

Temperature and relative humidity will be logged using a HOBO® brand temperature and relative humidity logging instrument manufactured by Onset Computer Corporation (or equivalent) and will be set to collect data at five minute intervals. Data will be collected during the site visits for a minimum of 5 minutes before and 5 minutes after the collection of the formaldehyde sample at each trailer. Data logs will be divided into individual logs for each sample. A suggested method for this is to flag the start and stop times by an event marker at the start and finish of data collection. Data will be downloaded to a laptop at end of each day. Files will be labeled with site #, date, and visit number in a standard form. Data event flags will be confirmed on the sample collection data sheet. Files will be e-mailed each day to the database manager.

Data Sheets

Data sheets will be filled out prior to and during site visit. Information about trailer received prior to site visit will be confirmed at time of site visit. Data sheets will be faxed or sent overnight each day to the database manager.

SAMPLING STANDARD OPERATING PROCEDURE

Preparation prior to site visit:

Formaldehyde

Operational Checks:

1) Pump and calibrator batteries checked for charge and functionality.
2) Pump flow rates calibrated to 500 ± 50 milliliters per minute.
3) Sample tubes lot # and expiration date checked.
   (Expired tubes will be discarded)

4) If necessary, collect media blanks and label.
5) Stock coolers with "Blue Ice"
6) Sample tubes placed in cooler in number to be equal to trip blanks and samples to be collected + 2.

Temperature and Relative Humidity

Turn on HOBO® instrument and check for proper operation.

Operational checks:

1) Confirmation of time synchronization
   a) Time must agree ± 1 minute with Formaldehyde Chronometer.
   b) Time should be adjusted if necessary.
2) Confirm readings of HOBO® meet manufacturer's specifications.
   a) Temperature readings must be ± 0.63° C of average temperature reading of all HOBO® instruments in group.
   b) Humidity readings must be ± 2.5% of average humidity reading of all HOBO® instruments in group.
   c) Any HOBO® falling outside the manufacturer's specifications will be flagged as out of calibration and removed from service until a calibration is performed.
3) Confirm that HOBO® is set to log Temperature and Humidity measurements at five minute intervals.
   a) Adjust to 5 minute data logging interval if necessary.
   b) Confirm event marker is operating correctly. (If not remove from service)

Data Sheet

10. Confirm information is correct for scheduled site visits.
11. Confirm sheets for all scheduled site visits are present.

Site Visit:

Formaldehyde

1. Calibrate pumps to a flow rate of 500 ± 50 milliliters per minute.
2. Record pump identification and pre-sample flow rate data on data sheet.
3. Label Sample tube.
4. Sample tube and trip blank data recorded on data sheet.
5. Sample tube set on tripod at central unobstructed location in the THU at breathing level.
6. Pump started and time recorded on data sheet.
7. Sample collected for 60 ± 2 minutes.
8. Pump stopped sample immediately capped and stop time recorded on data sheet.
9. Sample returned to cooler.
10. Pump post sample flow rate checked and recorded on data sheet.
11. Sample identification on tube confirmed with data on sample sheet.
12. Trip blanks will be recorded, processed, labeled and returned to cooler.

Temperature and Relative Humidity

1. Confirm that data logger is operating.
    a. LED blinks.
2. Activate event marker at least 5 minutes prior to start of formaldehyde sample.
    a. Press button for one second.
3. Record start time for HOBO® sample on data sheet.
4. Continue sampling until at least 5 minutes after completion of Formaldehyde sample, activate event marker to indicate end time of data collection.
    a. Press button for one second
5. Record stop time on data sheet.

Data Sheet

1. Confirm with the occupants that information previously provided is correct
2. Completely fill out data sheet.
3. Have second team member confirm that data sheet is complete.

Post Site Visit:

Formaldehyde

Monday - Friday samples

1. Confirm that the proper numbers of field and media blanks are enclosed.
2. Chain of custody documents completed for each sample.
3. Cooler "Blue Ice" refreshed.
4. Cooler sealed and shipping label affixed for overnight shipment to lab.

Saturday and Sunday samples

1. Confirm that the proper numbers of field and media blanks are enclosed.
2. Chain of custody documents completed for each sample.
3. Samples stored in freezer.

Monday morning

1. Cooler "Blue Ice" refreshed.
2. Cooler sealed and shipping label affixed for overnight shipment to lab.

Temperature and Relative Humidity

1. Data downloaded to a laptop hard drive.
   a. Data files will be named with Site #, date and visit number in the form – LA 001.10-12-2007.01. (Or similar)
2. Data file event marks will be checked against data sheet start and stop times.
3. Data e-mailed to data base manager.

Data sheet

Fax or overnight data sheet to data base manager.

APPENDIX G:
SAMPLE DATA SHEET FOR FORMALDEHYDE, TEMPERATURE, AND
RELATIVE HUMIDITY DATA COLLECTION

Date _____ (mm/dd/yyyy)

Sampling Team _____

TRAILER INFORMATION

THU Manufacturer _____

THU Model _____

VIN Number _____

Unique Trailer ID _____

Date of Manufacture _____ (mm/dd/yyyy)

THU Address _____

THU Type   □ Travel trailer   □ Mobile home   □ Park   □ Other

Unit Faces: N   S   E   W   (circle one)

Neighborhood   North:
Residential/Office/Retail/Manufacturer/Other_____

South:
Residential/Office/Retail/Manufacturer/Other_____

East:
Residential/Office/Retail/Manufacturer/Other_____

West:
Residential/Office/Retail/Manufacturer/Other_____

Comments:

_____

_____

_____

_____

APPENDIX G, con't:
SAMPLE DATA SHEET

Date _____ (mm/dd/yyyy)

Sampling Team _____

TEMPERATURE and RELATIVE HUMIDITY

Sample Location   _____
Sampling Height (inches)   _____
HOBO No.   _____
HOBO S/N   _____
Start Time   _____ AM/PM   Stop Time   _____ AM/PM
HOBO Data File Name

_____

FORMALDEHYDE SAMPLE

Sample Number _____ _____		Tube Lot
Pump Number S/N _____ _____		Tube S/N
Pre-Sample Calibration Flow (LPM) _____ AM/PM		Start Time _____
Post-Sample Calibration Flow (LPM) _____ AM/PM		Stop Time _____
Average Flow (LPM) _____ _____		Sample Time (min)
Sample Volume (L) _____		
Field Blank S/N _____ #_____		Chain of Custody
Shipped via _____ _____		Shipping #

THU ENVIRONMENT DURING SAMPLING

Number of windows open:	❑ 0	❑ 1	❑ 2	❑ 3 ❑ 4
Door open?	❑ Yes	❑ No	❑ Don't know	
Air conditioning on?	❑ Yes	❑ No	❑ Don't know	
Heat on?	❑ Yes	❑ No	❑ Don't know	
Exhaust hatch open?	❑ Yes	❑ No	❑ Don't know	

Comments:

_____

_____

Corrections:

_____

_____

www.ingramcontent.com/pod-product-compliance
Lightning Source LLC
Chambersburg PA
CBHW081854170526
45167CB00007B/3013